The 40 Secrets of How to Perfect Smile Training

Extra skills frame the ancient East

Reading Smart Life eBook in an hour!

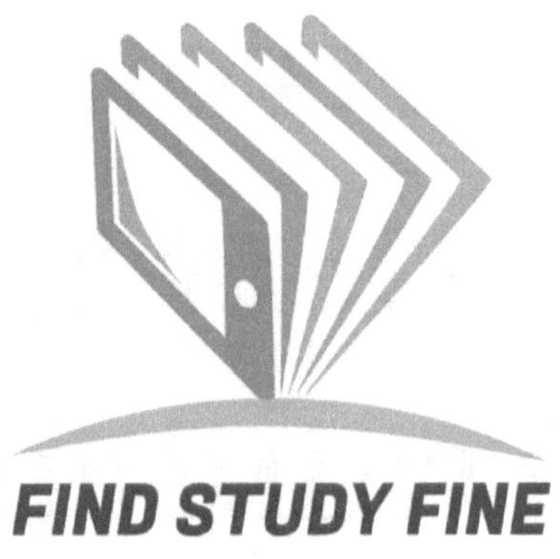

Copyright © 2018 by Find Study Fine Studio

Contents

Introduction

Have you been told by other people that you're laughing so poorly?

When you take self-portraits, do you always laugh unnaturally in the photo?

So don't you like to share your smiles or photos with everyone?

There are many muscles in the face as there are in the body. The activity of speaking and smiling makes use of only a small fraction of the muscles in the face- not more than about 30 percent. The muscles that are not in use begin to wane and fade away, especially as one begins to age. The truth of the matter is that a good smile makes one look years younger than his or her age because there is more use made of the muscles and for a longer period of time. This increases blood flow around the parts that make up the face, to keep that part healthy and youthful. However, there are special techniques that can be used both to get the facial expression that is required and to improve smile quality. The training makes the muscles flexible and not rigid, to make the smile natural and less of plastic. Some of these techniques are as follows to increasing smile quality.

Here we go!

Chapter 1

FACIAL MOVEMENT TO ELIMINATE PROLAPSE OF THE EYE

A smile includes the expression of the eyes. If the condition of the eye is not good, then the laugh will look unhappy and unnatural. So this is a key part of it that needs to be adjusted.

1. Squint movement

The drooping of eyelids sometimes makes a smile seem so unnatural. There is a practice called squint movement that helps to improve the quality of a smile. This consists of the opening of the mouth in the shape of the letter 'O' in a full way, and squint your eyes when there is bright light around. Do it in a repeated manner for 2-4 seconds. It has the effect of making the eyelid muscles to contract and relax at the same time. When it is done regularly, the quality of the resulting smile is greatly improved. Starts with 10 times a day, then increase it to around 100 times each day. It makes the lower eyelids to resume normally in their function after about two weeks of repeated exercise.

2. Open and close eyes

Another one is the open and close action of the eyes. Just do this five times, without pushing the eyes too hard, and without frowning. The skin in the middle of the eyes will swell, and in effect, you don't need to exercise the other muscles of the face.

3. Acupoint massage

When a massage is nicely done on the periphery of the eyes, it has a good effect on the quality of the smile that will result subsequently. It has to be gently done because of the fragile nerves. It is called acupoint massage. It has to be done gently or else there will be wrinkles around the eyes. It removes and stops tiredness of the eyes and reduces eyelid relaxation as well. Eye creams are also helpful in this regard. It is used to relieve fatigue around the eyes and bulging of the skin around the eyes.

Massaging the following eye points should create a positive feeling.

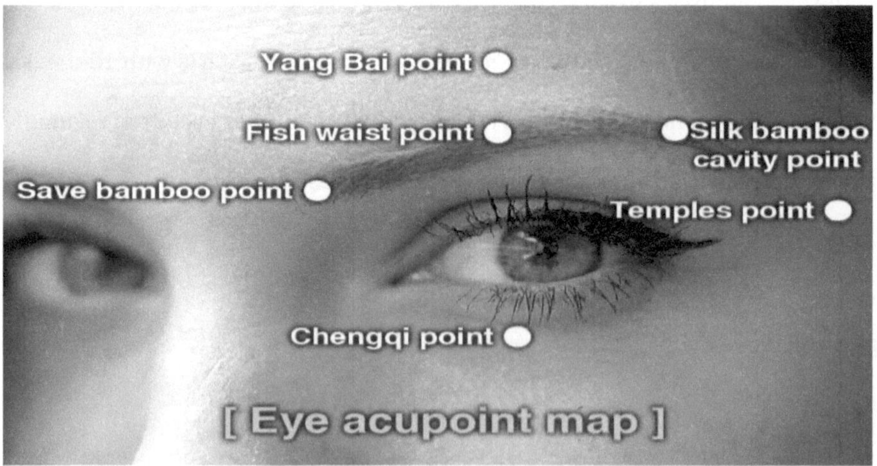

(a) Save Bamboo Point: Located at the lower part of the eyebrow, this point helps in the relieving of eye fatigue, headaches and swellings around the eyes.

(b) Fish Waist Point: This is located in the middle of the eyebrow and helps in reducing eye fatigues when massaged.

(c) Yang Bai Point: Located on the forehead, directly above the pupil, just above the midpoint of the eyebrow, it helps in reducing headaches.

(d) Silk Bamboo Cavity Point: Located at the end of the eyebrow, massaging this point can help to eliminate eye fatigue.

(e) Temples Point: This is located at the side of the head just beside the tip of the eyebrow and outermost corner of the eyes. This point helps in relieving eye fatigue and swelling.

(f) Chengqi Point: With the eyes looking directly forward, the point is located just below the pupil between the eyeball and infra-orbital ridge.

Chapter 2

ELIMINATION OF NASOLABIAL FOLD AND FACIAL MUSCLE MOVEMENT

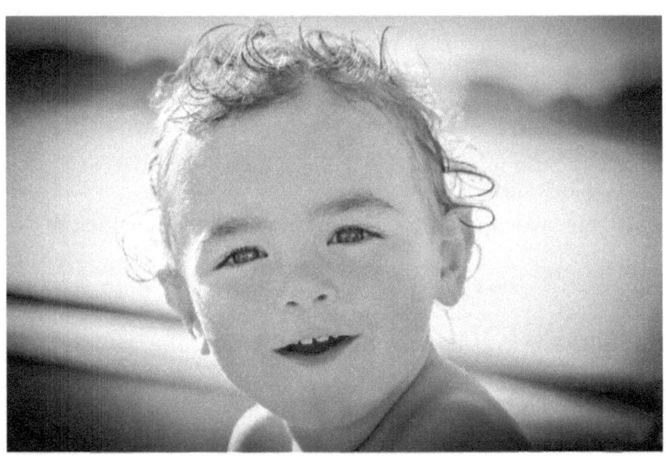

Having a very obvious nasolabial fold will often make a person look angry, even if that was not what was intended. So repairing your nasolabial fold is also an important part.

4. Reduce the use of computer or mobile phone

The use of computers or cell phones for prolonged periods of time causes a sagged skin around the face. This is because the use of the phone or computer makes you look downwards and maintain it for a long period and your countenance will always be expressionless. The facial muscles become inured to this posture and find it difficult to shift ground when you want to smile, making it very awkward looking. So in effect, reduce the amount of time spent on the phone and computer.

5. Suck the air

An exercise called the swollen double cheek movement has the potential of relaxing the cheek muscles and prevents falling out of place of the face. This is best done when you feel that your cheeks feel dull. The procedure is done by blowing the cheeks and filling it for about 10seconds. Suck the air back into the mouth and remain that way for the same amount of time. It can be repeated for a number of times.

6. Movement of the tongue and lips

This technique was invented by Ninjas during the warring state period of Japan to fight off halitosis. Not only can you eliminate bad breath with this method, but you can also prevent stripes. Here is a two-step process on how to perform this technique.

(a) Keep your lips closed and move your tongue around your mouth, in all directions.

(b) Move your tongue twice in one direction and twice in the other direction and the move it all over you mouth in all directions up to 4 times. Repeat these two steps up to 5 times.

7. Mouth practice:

(a) Start by opening your mouth as wide as you can. In doing so, your mouth will suddenly start shrinking and becoming smaller. Repeat this step 5 times.

(b) Widen one corner of your mouth to the right for 5 seconds.

(c) Do the same with the other corner of your mouth but to the left this time around for same 5 seconds. Repeat this step 5 times.

8. Corner of the mouth:

Start by stretching your throat and protruding your chin forward. Then fold your lower lip over the upper lip and raise your mouth. Do this once in the morning for 5mins and once in the evening for 5mins as well.

9.   Eating hard food:

Eating hard food requires us to chew with more energy and in doing so, we actually end up training the muscles near the mouth. Ensure you chew your food properly during breakfast, lunch and dinner. Chew with both your right and left side to prevent drooping of the chin.

Chapter 3

HEAD AND NECK EXERCISE

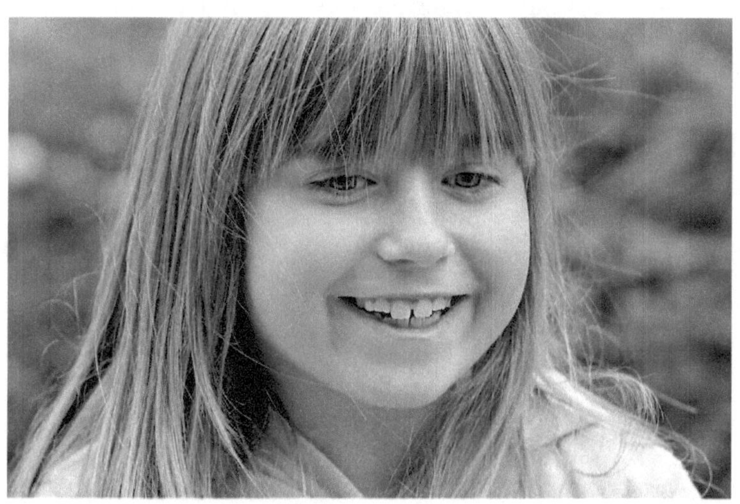

If the neck muscles are stiff, the blood supply towards the face and head becomes insufficient and this can result in the smile looking very stiff. This exercise is done mainly to make the neck muscles more flexible, not only to the eye training and the turning smile to help, but also to health benefits.

10. Head exercise

(a) The first step requires you to stand up or sit up and gently turn your neck to the left, return it back to normal, turn to the right and return it back to normal. Keep doing this repeatedly until satisfied.

(b) The second step is the front and back position which entails moving your head down, return it back to normal, move it up and return back. Do this continuously until satisfied.

(c) The third step involves gently rotating the neck in a continuous manner. This is done to make the neck muscles more flexible.

11. Neck muscle strength training

(a) Resistance Lateral Bending: Sit upright, place your right palm above your right ear, tilt your head to the right while the right hand offers support to keep your head in place. Do this for 5 seconds. Carry out the same process for the left hand and left ear. Ten times each for both sides.

(b) Resistance Forward Motion: Sit upright, place your forehead on your palm then apply pressure on the palm to keep the head in place. Maintain this position for 5 seconds. This can be repeated up to 10 times.

Chapter 4

FACIAL MASSAGE

The major aim of this step is to broaden the facial muscles so as to bring out an exceptional beauty when smiling.

12. Cream massage by nasolabial fold

(a) During the daily use of facial skin care cream, take two fingers full of cream on both hands. Using the index and middle finger, place the cream evenly on both sides of the nose. This is the starting point of the nasolabial fold.

(b) Use both the index and middle finger to rub from both sides of the nose to under the lip in a circular motion to help the skin absorb the cream and also to stimulate the skin in order to get rid of wrinkles.

(c) Slide the middle and index finger in the direction of the lips as if to pull up the sides of the mouth. Doing this helps in avoiding slacks on the lips.

(d) Gently apply pressure to the two corners of the nose and also the outermost part of the lips. This should be repeated up to 5 times to allow the skin totally ingest the cream. Concentrate on the pressure and try not to put too much force. This step is meant to be quite soothing.

13. Pressing the imaginary energy line with the index finger

This action will help smooth the wrinkles and nasolabial fold lines from the nose to the corner of the mouth, making it easier to laugh with smooth. Use of your imagination during the step will help enhance the impact of movement.

(a) While sitting, lay open your mouth and extend the upper lip above the upper row of teeth.

(b) Next, imagine a line of energy lowing from the corner of the mouth to the nostrils, moving downwards to the side of the mouth. Using the forefinger, move down that imaginary line in a repeated motion until the facial muscles feel sore. Afterwards, using only the upper and lower part of the index finger, press down 30 times. **Note**: Keep your face in step (a) when pressing down.

14. Whole facial massage

(a) As though covering your lips, lift your fingers up and move along the line to the sides of your nose.

(b) Continuously raise your forefinger to the sides of the nose.

(c) Move the fingers upwards to the inner corner and press for 35 seconds.

(d) Using the left hand, pull the left part of the cheek then use the right hand to push the right side of the face and also push the right cheek muscles to the corner of the eye for 3-5 seconds afterwards reduce pressure. Do this for the other side as well.

(e) Close your fingers together and start sliding you hand from the chin to the ear. Doing so will result in the whole face being pulled upwards. Then use the thumb and index finger to press on the face from the bottom to the top.

15. Pressing the highest point of the cheekbone

Widen both corners of your mouth and make a smile expression. As both corners of the mouth are stretched, press the highest point of the cheekbone with both hands. Do these up to 30 times as it can help improve the lines at the side of the mouth to the chin.

Chapter 5

Have you ever seen how unhappy you look when the muscles around your eyes don't move? Happiness can be seen in the eyes as well as a true smile. For instance, pretend you are smiling at a loved one or you have to take a picture smiling with the one you love. Your eyes will squint a bit with your lips slightly curved upwards and your smile will look really beautiful and more realistic.

To make your smile look more realistic, you should also add the effect of your eyes into the smile. A truly sincere smile is natural and real because it is difficult to use the muscles around your eyes except you really have something to be happy about.

Use eye skills to enhance the emotional expression of a smile, making it more attractive. The difference can be observed by making use of a mirror.

16. Squeeze your eyes:

Squeeze your eyes like you are about to squint. While doing that, let your eyelids sag then gently squint your eyes with a slight upwards curve on your lips without revealing your teeth. This is a subtle method of smiling with your eyes.

Smiling can express your friendliness and interest in a particular situation. Smiling makes people look more attractive and approachable because it shows confidence and it is also sexy. Scientists have discovered over 50 types of smile and the most sincere one of them all is the **DUCHENNE SMILE**. Although this might seem a bit cunning, but you can mimic this smile by gently squinting your eyes while observing it through a mirror. If you do have a bit of crow's feet (the muscle which contracts around the eyes resulting in the appearance of distinctive wrinkles) at the corner of your eyes, then you are doing the right thing.

Once you can learn how to smile with your eyes, you can even make a cunning and stiff smile look more beautiful. Every time you laugh, you must remember to squint your eyes no matter what but for some, it comes in naturally. However, try not to go too far, otherwise, your expression will become distorted. As long as you narrow your eyes, you should have a lovely smile. Keep eye contact with other people when you squint your eye as this will prove to be very effective.

17. Eyes only smile

Those who are really good at smiling can express happiness and joy without moving their mouths. This is not to say that you have to "keep your mouth shut", but when you smile with your eyes, try not to move your lips or grin as much as possible.

If you were successful in achieving the **DUCHENNE SMILE**, challenge yourself this time around in performing again but without the use of your lips. Training yourself to be highly skilled in smiling with just your eyes will help you to be able express bliss and joy without using your mouth to form a smile but at the same time, you don't have a frown up on your mouth as well. When trying to be mysterious, smiling with just the eyes can prove to be very useful. Smiling with the eyes can also be useful when you are trying not to fake a smile, as well as being in a situation where you are   trying to hold a nice expression.

18. Eye etiquette

Learn how to observe how people express their smile through their rich and colorful eyes. Pay full attention to eye etiquette. Do not look at strangers for a long period of time unless they appreciate it. Also, try not to blink too fast or too slow. Avoid using looks of contempt as well.

19. Imitating the eyes of animals

Male eyes are as strong as an eagle, which signifies perseverance while the eye of the female is more like that of a cat i.e. A phoenix. It portrays gentleness, kindness, agility and beauty. Using your eyes to express different emotions can make your smiles have different meanings.

Chapter 6

PRONUNCIATION AUXILLARY METHOD

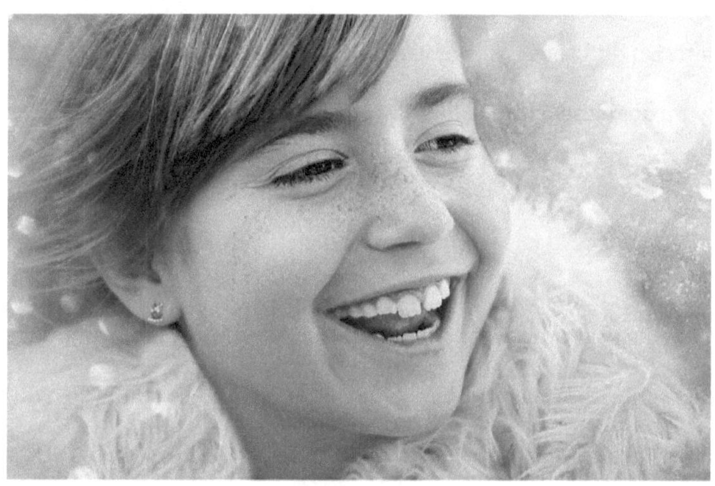

Through different pronunciations, one can not only adjust the shape of the mouth smile, but also train the whole oral movement coordination ability.

20. Do-Re-Mi. relaxation exercise

Relaxing the muscles around the lips is the first stage of the smile practice. The Do-Re-Mi exercise helps the lip muscles to relax. It begins with the bass and moves to the treble which helps in speaking loudly and should be done three times. This process however, is not a continuous practice but rather, a syllable to syllable pronunciation. In order to get the correct pronunciation, we should pay attention to the shape of the mouth during the pronunciation practice.

21. Similar pronunciation exercise

Making use of small mirror, observe your smiling face. Find the beautiful smiling pattern for yourself by using some similar accents or alphabetical pronunciations such as "E", "S", "ho", and "ha" etc. Do different types of training to make the facial muscles active and them full of elasticity through the expressions.

22. O & E exercises

(a) Using both hands, press the highest point of the cheekbone and pronounce the letter "O". With this same process, pronounce the letter "E" and by doing so, you will feel firmness in the face. You can do this up to 30 times with the alphabet "O" and "E".

(b) Press your middle finger on your cheek then use both your index and ring finger to form a stripe beside it as you pronounce the letter "O". Maintaining this same position, switch to the letter "E" and open your mouth as far as possible.

These two steps can be repeated 10 times each.

23. A E I O U exercises

Use the letters **A E I O U** to train the facial muscles. Each word should be said for at least 5 seconds. Sagging of the face can be reduced by repeatedly performing this exercise. This exercise works better when in a relaxed state, so it is advisable to perform it when in a bath or any other relaxed state you can think of.

24. Singing method

Beauty experts believe that singing is a cosmetic tool that allows rhythmic movement of facial muscles which promotes the supply of facial blood and increases the vitality of facial tissue cells as it makes the face brighter and more flexible. Psychologists believe that singing can regulate people's mood and can also cure diseases.

According to this, our brain thinks that both singing loudly or quietly is good for both the movement and the mood adjustment of the facial muscles and is also certainly good for the smile training. In this case, from the smile training point of view, it is advisable to smile both before and after singing.

Chapter 7

MOUTH SHAPE AUXILIARY METHOD

This is an auxiliary way to adjust the smile curve of the mouth, making the degree and goal of the smile clearer than before.

25. The stir bar or chopstick method

Place a small mirror in front of you and then proceed to examine your smiling face in front of it. Afterwards, follow the steps below:

(a) Take a stir bar or chopstick and place it in-between your upper and lower teeth.

(b) Both sides of the chopstick or stir bar (depending on which you decide to go for) should touch both side of your cheeks and also maintain its height.

(c) Carefully adjust the radian on both sides of your mouth as high as possible. This would be hard to achieve at first but continuous practice and training would make it easier over time. This helps in maintaining a longer smile.

(d) Maintain the previous step and remove the chopsticks. The corner of the mouth is the main factor when smiling. You should be able to see the eight teeth in the upper row of your mouth.

(e) Once again, bite down gently on the chop sticks and move the corner of your mouth upwards. Repeat this movement for 30 seconds.

(f) Remove the chopstick and notice your facial expression when you smile. Use your hands to hold up your cheeks and push them from bottom to top.

(g) Put down your hands and repeat steps (a, b, c & d) and try making a form of "E" sound as well. Repeat this for 30 seconds or more.

26. Dental exposure

Place a mirror in front of you and observe your face when you smile. A smile isn't meant to be bare as you are meant to show your teeth when smiling. Showing the upper teeth is for a light smile, showing the upper and lower eight teeth is for a middle laugh while opening your teeth to show your tongue is for a big laugh.

The most beautiful smile curve can be achieved by showing 6-8 teeth but take note that each individual has different teeth arrangement so you don not really have to take into consideration the amount of teeth being shown.

27. Gingiva (gum) practice

When smiling, confirm the number of gums you can see. If you desire to smile without exposing a lot of gum, probably seeing the gums within 2mm is pretty good, then give your upper lip a little more pressure and pull it down. Maintain this position for 10 seconds.

28. Double finger

Protrude your thumb and index finger as you gently clench the rest three fingers. Place the top of each thumb under the chin, place each of the index fingers at the side of the mouth then push gently. Do this repeatedly until satisfied.

OR

Extend both the thumb and forefinger while holding the rest fingers in place. Place the index fingers of both hands on the outer part of your two eye brows, place both of your thumbs at the corner of your mouth and gently pull. Repeat this process until you are satisfied.

29. Smile Facial Muscle Exerciser

Some "netizens" confirmed that after the use of Smile Facial Muscle Exerciser for a week, their smiles have become much better than before. But, some "netizens" also claimed that it do not have any result on them. There are many kinds of Smile Facial Muscle Exercisers which you can buy in the market but there is no certain result.

Chapter 8

IDEA ASSISTANT METHOD

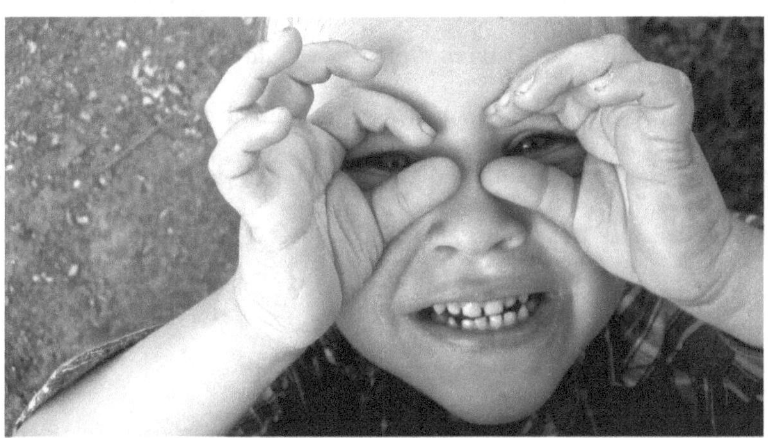

The following methods are a little bit difficult. These are based on the above mentioned methods but then then use your mind to improve them. Most of them are the East techniques

30. Mindfulness

This is a form of training that is the higher form of smiling. Instead of looking into the mirror or other surfaces, you can make use of your mind to control and move your lips to achieve your best smile. This step has a lot of benefits which includes:

- You don't have to use a mirror
- You can do it quietly at any time and place plus it is the best way to develop a sense of smile.

31. Memory retrieval

Get together with a few friends and share a few laughs with them. Pay close attention to how you smile in this moment when you are truly happy, save it up in your memory then later, try reliving his moments in mind. Doing so should trigger how you felt back then which should produce a genuine smile. This is a method commonly used by actors in training known as Emotional Memory Method. It brings your happiest memories back to life in your mind which causes you to smile again. Observe and compare which smile is the most beautiful and genuine smile.

32. Guide smile training

Place a small mirror in front of you and observe your smile on it.

(a) Close your lips.

(b) Point the forefinger of both hands towards each other, and then proceed to placing them 15 to 20 centimeters in front of the mouth.

(c) Move the tips of both fingers to the left and right at a slow constant pace till they are 5 to 10 millimeters apart. Doing so would create a beautiful smile.

(d) Move the two index fingers towards the middle at a slow steady pace until they both meet. At the same time, the corners of the smiling lips would slowly begin to retract. It is crucial to note that the smile is now slowly held back. Do not let the smile stop all of a sudden. Carry out this training at least 30 times.

33. Find a true smile

Pay attention to your facial expression and how you feel whenever you smile. For example, if someone makes you laugh due to a funny joke, ask yourself these questions to help you remember what a real smile feels like.

- What makes you smile when you go through your memories? Try to reproduce that feeling.
- What was the position of you five senses? Take a look in the mirror before the smile disappears and focus on what your real smile looks like.

34. Habit of fake laughter

People going through a tough time at work or in life tend to wrap it all up in form of a fake smile which thus, embodies the positive role of the fake laugh. Forcing yourself to forget your worries and pretending to smile can change the state of your mind and the state of your natural smile. Finally, your smirk will become a real smile.

35. Have happy triggers ready

It is important to create happy triggers or habits that would aid in tour smiling skills seeing as you won't always be happy during your daily activities. When creating a trigger, keep in mind that is has to be something you experience daily without you having to search through your memory to remember. For example:

- If you happen to be giving a speech or a presentation, train yourself to automatically place a smile, each time you turn to the next page of your presentation or the next paragraph of your speech,

- Words can also be used as triggers. In such a manner that anytime you hear certain words, you automatically smile. These words could be anything, depending on you. It could even be the word "and". Find a word that suits you or a word you hear often.

Chapter 9

GROUP ASSISTANT METHOD

Practice all the smiling methods individually, and finally use them flexibly in the group to make them more proficient and flawless.

36. The guide of others

Create a training environment with friends. Find some interesting materials, try to make each other laugh and share the skills and experience of how to smile. Most of your shortcomings need to be seen through the eyes of others so they can give you feedback. This is a great way to make progress quickly.

37. Specific social environment training

Meeting new people as well as familiar faces can help you know how best to place your smile. Communicate with people of various age groups, sexes, professions and personalities in different situations and try making use of different smiling methods to see the effect it has on them.

Chapter 10

SMILE TABOO

38. Avoid excessive laughter

Laughing too much can result in having an excessive grin which can make one feel silly. The best way to overcome this effect is having an honest frame of mind. You do not have to force yourself to laugh way more than what you actually feel.

39. Slow down your smile

Learn how to slow down your smile instead of suddenly stopping the smile. Doing so without any warning would have a negative effect.

40. Restrained smile

A restrained smile can help show your beauty. Laughing for a really short period of time or for a really long period of time isn't so good, so try avoiding that at all costs. For example, you work at a shop, when interacting with customers, funny topics tend to come up so it is advisable to place just a smile instead of using excessive laughter.

CONCLUSION

Despite the fact that there is a lot of serious training required to correct and achieve a glorious smile, if the smile isn't perfect in the end, it is important to find other parts of what might have caused this. But if we can laugh confidently, we can turn failures into satisfaction and not difficulties. For example,

- When the corner of the mouth rises, it becomes crooked and when this happens, the use of chopsticks for training would prove to be very effective. Although it may be hard at first but with constant practice, the corners of the mouth will unconsciously start to rise on both sides thereby forming a capable and sophisticated smile.

- When laughing, people who show too much gum often smile with little or no confidence. It is usually more of a shy smile. Smiling naturally can make up for the "downside" of too much gum showing but due to lack of confidence, they find it hard to laugh naturally. When the gums are exposed, the muscles are trained to compensate for the too much of exposure.

Combine all four elements to achieve the perfect smile.

(a) The combination of mouth and eyes to be eloquent and smiling to actually express your heart and how you feel.

(b) Laugh and character combined. The soul makes the smile filled with emotions. 'Love' makes the laugh filled with feelings, kindness, sweetness, and reflects the beautiful heart while character, keeping in mind that it is a good character, makes the laugh filled with humility, stability, generosity and decentness.

(c) Combine laughter with language. Both language and smile are very important for the dispersion of information so it is important to pay attention to both of these

(d) Let your smile be combined with culture, etiquette and manners to help you laugh properly.

Finally, choose your preferred method above and every morning of everyday, train as soon as you wake up for as long as you can till you are finally able to achieve that perfect smile.

Before stepping out each day, say to yourself "Today is a beautiful day and you are really happy".

Make smiling a habit.

Recommended Books:

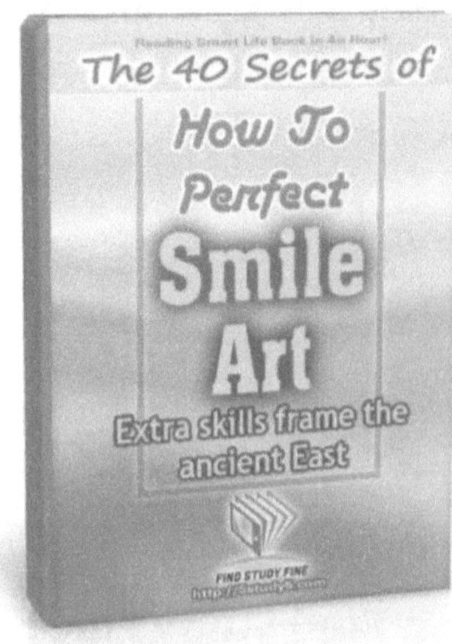

Preview the Book "The 40 Secrets of How to Perfect Smile Art"

- Owing to changing times and the creeping up of negativity in the world, there have come to be less and less reason to smile.
- The solution is to always be your own cheerleader, whether someone else joins you or not.
- Dress sense is another key way of increasing your confidence and adding to you many more reasons to smile.
- When that is done, confidence is restored and the smile is more constant and deep.

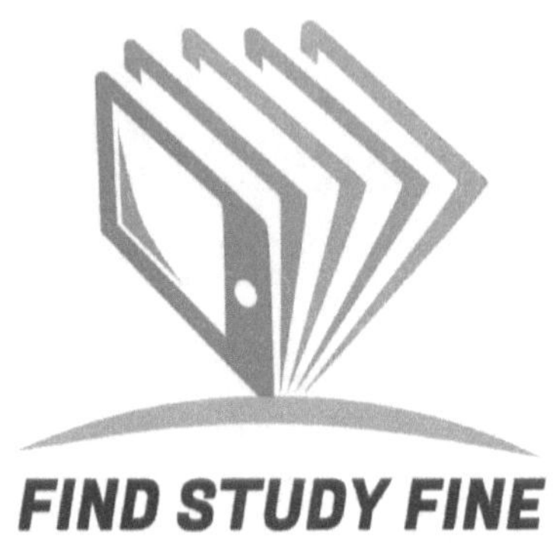

About Find Study Fine Studio

Our studio is committed to improving the lives of everyone, creating rich content and presenting it in the most important way.

We spend a lot of time making great products and you can learn all the key points and tips in the shortest time from us.

Find Study Fine Studio is your best learning friend!

Before you leave, I wanted to say thank you again for reading our book.

Have a nice day!